Catherine Cavallaro Goodman, M.B.A., P.T.
Formerly, Visiting Assistant Professor, Clinical Director
University of Montana
Missoula, Montana
Private Practice
Missoula, Montana

Teresa E. Kelly Snyder, M.N., R.N., C.S.
(Clinical Specialist in Medical-Surgical Nursing)
Associate Professor of Nursing
Montana State University
Bozeman, Montana

▪ ▪ ▪ ▪ ▪ ▪ ▪ ▪ ▪ ▪ ▪

Differential Diagnosis in Physical Therapy

SECOND EDITION

W.B. SAUNDERS COMPANY
A Division of Harcourt Brace & Company
Philadelphia London Toronto Montreal Sydney Tokyo

W.B. SAUNDERS COMPANY
A Division of Harcourt Brace & Company

The Curtis Center
Independence Square West
Philadelphia, Pennsylvania 19106

Library of Congress Cataloging-in-Publication Data

Goodman, Catherine Cavallaro.
   Differential diagnosis in physical therapy / Catherine Cavallaro Goodman,
Teresa E. Kelly Snyder.—2nd ed.

   p.   cm.

   Includes bibliographical references and index.

   ISBN 0–7216–5267–0

   1. Physical therapy. 2. Diagnosis, Differential. I. Snyder, Teresa E.
Kelly. II. Title
   [DNLM: 1. Physical Therapy 2. Diagnosis, Differential. WB 460
G653d 1994]

   RM701.G66   1995   616.07′5—dc20

   DNLM/DLC   93-49789

Differential Diagnosis in Physical Therapy   ISBN 0–7216–5267–0
2nd edition

Printed in the United States of America

Last digit is the print number: 9   8   7   6   5   4   3   2   1

To Cliff, Ben, and Guy,
who have finally pulled themselves together
and made this second edition possible.
C.C.G.

To my husband, R.C.; my son, Jim; and my daughter, Deann,
who fill my life with laughter and enthusiasm
T.E.K.S.

Foreword

■ ■ ■ ■ ■ ■ ■ ■ ■ ■ ■

This book is an invaluable resource for responsible physical therapy practice. Goodman and Snyder have presented in a clear and concise manner the information needed to screen patients for medical conditions. In addition, the processes of history taking and decision making they describe provide a good model to aid therapists in developing diagnostic skills.

A major change in physical therapy practice over the past 30 years has been the amount of responsibility assumed by physical therapists. Thirty years ago most physical therapists treated hospital inpatients, with physicians and nurses nearby to closely monitor the patients' medical conditions during physically demanding rehabilitation. Today fewer physical therapists work in hospitals, and current trends suggest that those numbers will continue to diminish. More physical therapists are working in settings without physicians, such as nursing homes, outpatient clinics, and patients' homes. The patients in these settings can be more seriously ill than those formerly treated in hospitals, and thus their medical conditions require greater monitoring.

Present efforts at cost containment suggest that referred patients will have less-extensive diagnostic testing than they had in the past. In addition, more than half the states allow patients to receive physical therapy without a referral and thus without examination by a physician. Physical therapists have always had the responsibility of recognizing unreported symptoms or medical conditions that preclude treatment. However, the likelihood of physical therapists' encountering such conditions is much greater now than it has ever been. When establishing a patient's movement impairment diagnosis, the physical therapist must understand the difference between movement disorders and the diseases or pathologies diagnosed by physicians. Because many impairments are consequences of disease, the physical therapist should identify and recognize conditions requiring a diagnosis by a physician.

The authors' experience as direct-contact practitioners, responsible for medical screening, explains the appropriateness of the text to the needs of physical therapists. The purpose of this text is not to have physical therapists make a differential medical diagnosis; that is beyond their scope of practice. Rather, the intention is to describe the medical conditions whose symptoms mimic musculo-skeletal problems; knowing these conditions is critical for safe practice. Goodman and Snyder have written a well-organized and timely book. This book contains vital information physical thera-pists need for responsible patient care and should be a welcome resource for many other nonphysician clinicians.

SHIRLEY A. SAHRMANN, PH.D., P.T., F.A.P.T.A.
Associate Professor of Physical Therapy/Neurology
Director, Movement Science Program
Washington University School of Medicine
St. Louis, Missouri

Preface

Since publication of the first edition of *Differential Diagnosis in Physical Therapy*, the need for medical screening of all physical therapy clients has become readily apparent. Increased specialization in the health care delivery system combined with new and more virulent diseases has resulted in both a "sicker" client base and an increased possibility that systemic conditions will mimic musculoskeletal signs and symptoms.

In today's technically oriented research era, information about diseases and medical treatment is constantly changing. These advances are especially true in the areas of cardiology, organ transplants, oncology, and disease entities such as tuberculosis, human immunodeficiency virus (HIV), viral hepatitis, Lyme disease, Sjögren's syndrome, and others. The second edition incorporates this new information.

This edition also includes changes that reflect the need of students and clinicians for more information about systemic diseases that can present as musculoskeletal conditions. Whenever possible, information about disease etiology, risk factors, pathogenesis, and prognosis and treatment has been added to.

Summaries at the end of the chapters have been replaced with Key Points to Remember, which include composite illustrations of referred pain patterns associated with diseases in each organ system. Each chapter in the first edition had one case study to help the reader integrate the information presented into clinical practice; additional case examples have been added throughout each chapter.

Consumers of health care services are no longer viewed by clinical practitioners as passive recipients of treatment, referred to as "patients," but are encouraged as "clients" to participate in their own health care plan whenever possible. This change in nomenclature in current clinical practice is reflected in this second edition.

CATHERINE CAVALLARO GOODMAN

Acknowledgments

■ ■ ■ ■ ■ ■ ■ ■ ■ ■

Differential Diagnosis in Physical Therapy is a direct result of experience in the military as an independent practitioner over a period of 7 years. In addition to the numerous men and women of the United States Army who have assisted in bringing this book to publication, special thanks go to:

Steven Stratton, Ph.D., for the introduction to knowledge of systemic origins of neuromusculoskeletal disorders.

Maureen Fleming, Ph.D., and Ray Murray, Ph.D., for advice and counsel from the start and throughout this project.

Dorothy Patent, Ph.D., for her help and guidance in getting this book off the ground.

The physicians in our community, including Charles E. Bell, Thomas D. Bell, David W. Burgan, J. A. Cain, C. Paul Loehnen, C. Byron Olson, Dean E. Ross, Peggy Schlesinger, Stephen F. Speckart, John R. Stone, Nicholas R. Williams, and Wesley W. Wilson.

Robert C. Morgan, P.T., Ph.D., Chairman, Duquesne University Physical Therapy Program, for all the constructive criticism and helpful suggestions he has made toward this second edition.

Gene Mead, Ph.D., for keeping us up to date on the subject of acquired immunodeficiency syndrome (AIDS).

The staff of St. Patrick's Medical Library, especially Kim Granath, Medical Librarian, and Barb McFaden, for the numerous times that they provided help and information at the last minute.

Erling Oelz, Director of Public Service, University of Montana, Mansfield Library, for his help in staying abreast of current medical literature using CD-ROM and Medline.

The many authors and publishers who have allowed us to publish some of their tables and drawings in order to help present the information in a quick reference format for both students and physical therapy clinicians.

William Bailey, P.T., for permission to reproduce the case study in Chapter 2.

Margaret Biblis, Shirley Kuhn, and the staff of W. B. Saunders Company for their suggestions in writing this textbook.

To these people and to the many others who remain unnamed, we say thank you. Your support and encouragement have made *Differential Diagnosis in Physical Therapy* possible.

CATHERINE CAVALLARO GOODMAN
TERESA E. KELLY SNYDER

Contents

4
Overview of Pulmonary Signs and Symptoms 147

8

Overview of Hepatic and Biliary Signs and Symptoms......284

9

Overview of Endocrine and Metabolic Signs and Symptoms......325

10
Overview of Oncologic Signs and Symptoms 387

11
Overview of Immunologic Signs and Symptoms 452

12
Systemic Origins of Musculoskeletal Pain: Associated Signs and Symptoms 522

1

Introduction to Differential Screening in Physical Therapy

■ ■ ■ ■ ■ ■ ■ ■ ■ ■ ■

Clinical Signs and Symptoms of:

Panic Disorder
Depression

Whether following the model of independent practice under the increasingly prevalent direct access laws or practicing by physician referral, physical therapists must know how to recognize systemic disease masquerading as neuromusculoskeletal dysfunction.

Under direct access, the physical therapist may have primary responsibility or become the first contact for some clients in the health care delivery system. On the other hand, clients may obtain a signed prescription for physical therapy from their primary care physician, based on similar past complaints of musculoskeletal symptoms, without actually seeing that physician.

Additionally, with the increasing specialization of medicine, more and more clients are being evaluated for the first time by a medical specialist who may not recognize the underlying systemic disease. Lastly, early signs and symptoms of systemic disease may be difficult or impossible to recognize until the disease has progressed. In such cases, the alert physical therapist may be the first to ask the client pertinent questions to elicit underlying symptoms requiring medical referral.

It is important that physical therapists know when and how to refer clients to the appropriate health care practitioner. Such referral depends on the clinician's ability to quickly recognize problems that are beyond physical therapy expertise through knowledge of hallmark signs and symptoms of systemic illness.

Knowing that systemic diseases can mimic neuromusculoskeletal dysfunction, the physical therapist is responsible for identifying as closely as possible what neuromusculoskeletal pathology is present. This process includes investigating the possibility of systemic disease and determining the need for medical referral. The final result should be to treat as specifically as possible by closely identifying the underlying movement dysfunction and neuromusculoskeletal pathology.

By the end of your course of study of this material, you will know what questions to ask clients so that you can identify the need for medical referral, and you will know what medical conditions can cause shoulder, back, thorax, hip, sacroiliac, and groin pain.

This text provides students and physical therapy clinicians alike with a step-by-step approach to client evaluation, which follows the standards for competency established by the American Physical Therapy Association (APTA) related to conducting a screening examination. With the physical therapy interview as a foundation for subjectively evaluating each client, each organ system is reviewed with regard to the most common disorders encountered, particularly those that may mimic primary musculoskeletal lesions.

To assist the physical therapist in making a treatment-versus-referral decision, specific pain patterns corresponding to systemic diseases are presented. Special follow-up questions are listed in the subjective examination to help the physical therapist determine when these pain patterns are accompanied by associated signs and symptoms that indicate visceral involvement.

Throughout the text, guidelines for when and how to refer a client to a physician (or other health care provider) for further evaluation or medical follow-up are provided. Each individual case must be reviewed carefully. The client's history, presenting pain patterns, and possible associated signs and symptoms must be reviewed along with results from the objective evaluation in making a treatment-versus-referral decision.

PHYSICAL THERAPY DIAGNOSIS

Diagnosis is the recognition of disease. It is the determination of the cause and nature of pathologic conditions. Differential diagnosis is the comparison of symptoms of similar diseases so that a correct assessment of the client's actual problem can be made.

Diagnosis is also the name given to a collection of relevant signs and symptoms and names the primary dysfunction toward which the physical therapist directs treatment. The dysfunction is identified by the physical therapist based on the information obtained from the history, signs, symptoms, examination, and tests the therapist performs or requests. The function of a diagnosis is to provide information that can guide treatment (Sahrmann, 1988), and we must establish a diagnosis in a way that allows us to intervene within our legal scope of practice (Rose, 1989).

According to Rothstein (1993), in many fields of medicine when a diagnosis is made the pathologic condition is determined, and in addition, stages and classifications that guide treatment are named. We would do well to follow this model. We recognize that the term "diagnosis" relates to pathology, but we know that pathology alone is inadequate to guide the physical therapist (Rothstein, 1993). Classification schemes and categories are being discussed within our profession to enable us to make meaningful comparisons (Delitto et al. 1993; Magistro et al., 1993; Rothstein, 1993).

In 1984, the House of Delegates of the APTA passed the following motion: *"Physical therapists may establish a diagnosis within the scope of their knowledge, experience, and expertise"* (APTA, 1984).

In 1990, the Commission on Accreditation in Physical Therapy Education adopted Evaluative Criteria for Accreditation of Education Programs for the Preparation of Physical Therapists. In 1992, these accreditation standards became effective:

4.1.3. *The program graduates determine in any patient with physical therapy dysfunction a diagnosis that is within the scope of physical therapy by:*
    4.1.3.1. obtaining pertinent history and identifying patient problems through interview or other appropriate means
    4.1.3.2. selecting and performing appropriate examinations and interpreting the results of physical therapy examinations . . . (p.11)

The key phrase in these standards is *within the scope of physical therapy.* In making a diagnosis, physical therapists should confine themselves to neuromusculoskeletal lesions. As specialists in this field, physical therapists are usually able to make far more accurate diagnoses than most medical practitioners (McKenzie, 1981).

Physical therapists are required daily to make decisions regarding what they are educated, trained, and licensed to provide —that is, physical therapy evaluation and treatment (APTA, 1990). These decisions usually involve a determination of the location, severity, and treatment of a neuromusculoskeletal abnormality.

Identification of causative factors or etiology by the physical therapist is limited primarily to those pathokinesiologic problems associated with faulty biomechanical or neuromuscular action. (Pathokinesiology refers to the study of movements related to a given disorder.) Sahrmann (1988) noted that physical therapists' primary responsibility has been to understand anatomy and the components of kinesiology and pathokinesiology because this information is the basis of their practice.

Within this context, physical therapists communicate with physicians and other health care practitioners to request or recommend further medical evaluation. Additionally, whether in a private practice or in a home health, acute care hospital, or rehabilitation setting, physical therapists may observe some important finding outside the realm of neuromusculoskeletal disorders requiring additional medical evaluation and treatment.

Direct Access

Prior to 1968, a physician's referral was necessary for a client to be treated by a physical therapist. Now, more than half of the states in the United States permit direct access to physical therapy (APTA, 1990). The Physical Therapy Practice Act is being changed in many more states to provide for the independent practice of physical therapists. Thus, a consumer (i.e., the patient or client) can be evaluated and treated by a physical therapist in those states with direct access without previous examination of that client by a physician or other practitioner and subsequent referral to a physical therapist.

Independent practice requires that the physical therapist be able to evaluate a client's complaint knowledgeably and determine whether the client has signs and symptoms of a systemic disease or a medical condition that should be evaluated by a more appropriate health care provider. This text endeavors to provide the necessary information that will assist the physical therapist in making these decisions. The competencies for the physical therapy screening examination established by the APTA in 1985 and adopted in 1990 have been used to prepare this information.

The purpose and the scope of this text are not to teach physical therapists to be all-purpose diagnosticians. The concern for physical therapists in relation to direct access to clients is in the differentiation of clients who need an appropriate referral. The purpose of this text is to provide a method for physical therapists to recognize readily (in a step-by-step problem-solving manner) areas that are beyond their expertise.

DECISION-MAKING PROCESS

This text is designed to help physical therapists (as primary practitioners) to make appropriate decisions about treatment for the client. To help physical therapists with those important decisions, these four parameters are used in evaluating each client:

- **Client History** (Chapter 2)
- **Pain Patterns/Pain Types** (Chapter 1)
- **Systems Review** (Chapter 12)
- **Signs and Symptoms of Systemic Diseases** (Chapter 12)

This text includes the following features to assist the therapist in using all four parameters effectively:

- Diagnostic physical therapy interviewing
- Special features that include drawings of primary and referred pain patterns for quick reference
- Disease processes that mimic the pain of musculoskeletal disorders
- Dual representation of signs and symptoms by the system and by the anatomic part

The text has an active participatory focus, with emphasis on interacting and on speaking with the client and also on making treatment decisions. The following standards are within the competencies of APTA (1985) for conducting a screening examination:

Describe the clinical manifestations of the more common disorders of organ systems other than neuromuscular system(s).

Describe the etiology and clinical manifestations of disorders that mimic dysfunction of the neuromuscular system.

Describe normal and abnormal reactions to common drugs; drugs that may affect the neuromusculoskeletal system(s); drug reactions that mimic disorders of these systems and drug interactions.

Interpret information from the client's history, including a history that includes the client's description and perception of the chief complaint, an accurate and comprehensive medical and family/social history, and a comprehensive and appropriately focused review of organ systems.

Interpretation of the client's history must be accurate, identify noncontributory information, identify chief and secondary problems, identify information that is inconsistent with the presenting complaint, generate a working hypothesis regarding possible causes of complaints, and determine whether referral or consultation is indicated.

Client History (Diagnostic Interviewing)

The interview with the client is very important because it helps the physical therapist distinguish between problems that he or she can treat and problems that should be referred to a physician for diagnosis and treatment. This information establishes a solid basis for the physical therapy objective evaluation, assessment, and therefore treatment.

This material is intended to serve as a reference guide for the skilled clinician and as a teaching text for use with physical therapy students. The student of physical therapy can use the book to develop necessary skills for clinical work, and the experienced clinician can refer to it as a guide for addressing specific clinical issues.

For example, a student can use the detailed step-by-step breakdown of the interview with the client to understand and practice each part of the process. The experienced clinician can refer to chapters on systemic problems and can have access to information about what specific questions to address to each client, depending on the presenting chief complaint. For example, the person with chest pain should be asked specifically about both systemic and musculoskeletal origins of the present pain and symptoms.

An interviewing process is described that includes concrete and structured tools and techniques for conducting a thorough and informative interview. The use of follow-up questions is discussed because these questions help structure the interview.

Illiteracy

Throughout the interviewing process and even throughout the treatment period, the therapist must keep in mind that 25 million American adults are illiterate and an additional 35 million read only at a functional level for survival. In Boston, Massachusetts, 40 per cent of the adult population is illiterate. In San Antonio, Texas, 152,000 adults have been documented as illiterate, and over half the adult population in San Antonio alone is illiterate in English. Forty-four per cent of black adults are totally or partially illiterate, and 56 per cent of Hispanic adults are illiterate in English (Kozol, 1985).

These statistics do not take into account reading or learning disabilities. Functional literacy can vary depending on what the individual's need is, but in any case, having a reading level of fifth grade and below cannot help a person requiring care.

People who are illiterate cannot read instructions on bottles of prescription medicine or over-the-counter medications. They cannot know when a medicine is past the year of safe consumption, nor can they read about allergic risks, warnings to diabetics, or the potential sedative effect of medications. They cannot read about "the seven warning signs" of cancer or the indications of blood sugar fluctuations (Kozol, 1985). They cannot understand the written details on a health insurance form or read the details of exercise programs provided by physical therapists.

As with all sensitive areas, using a direct, professional approach is best when asking someone if he or she can read—for example:

As your physical therapist, I want to provide you with the best care possible. I often use written instructions for your use at home and I want to match these instructions to your needs. Can you read or would you prefer pictures only?

Case Studies

Case studies are provided with each chapter to provide the physical therapist with a working understanding of how to recognize the need for additional questions. In addition, information is given concerning the type of questions to ask and how to correlate the results with the objective findings. Whenever possible, information about when and how to refer a client to the physician is given. Each case study is based on actual case histories to provide reasonable examples of what to expect when the physical therapist is functioning as an independent practitioner who is the first health care provider to assess a client.

Pain Patterns/Pain Types

In each section, specific pain patterns characteristic of disease entities that can mimic pain from musculoskeletal disorders are discussed. Detailed information regarding the location, referral pattern, description, intensity, and duration of systemic pain is augmented by information about associated symptoms and relieving and aggravating factors. This information is compared with the presenting features of primary musculoskeletal lesions that have similar patterns of presentation.

Pain patterns of the chest, thoracic spine, shoulder, scapula, lumbar spine, groin, sacroiliac joint, and hip are included because these are the most frequent sites of referred pain from a systemic disease process.

Assessment of Pain and Symptoms

There are many possible *sources* of pain and many *types* of pain. Physical therapists frequently see clients whose primary complaint is pain, which often leads to a loss of function. Usually, a careful assessment of pain behavior is invaluable in determining the nature and extent of the underlying pathology. Development of an appropriate treatment program and evaluation of progress may depend mainly on an assessment of pain (Hertling and Kessler, 1990). Therefore, the portion of the core interview regarding a client's perception of pain is a critical factor in the evaluation of signs and symptoms.

The interviewing techniques and specific questions outlined in Chapter 2 result in a description of the client that is clear, accurate, and comprehensive. Questions must be understood by the client and should be presented in a nonjudgmental atmosphere. To elicit a more complete description of symptoms from the client, the physical therapist may wish to use a term other than "pain." For example, referring to the client's "symptoms" or using descriptors such as "hurt" or "sore" may be more helpful to some individuals (Jacox, 1977). If the client has completed the McGill Pain Questionnaire (Chapter 2), the physical therapist may choose the most appropriate alternative word selected by the client from the list to refer to the symptoms. The use of alternative words to describe a client's symptoms may also aid in refocusing attention away from pain and toward improvement of functional abilities.

SOURCES OF PAIN

In listening to the client's description of pain, four general sources of pain must be considered:

Cutaneous Pain (related to the skin). This source of pain includes superficial somatic structures located in the skin and subcutaneous tissue. The pain is well localized because the client can point directly to the area that "hurts." Cutaneous (skin) tenderness may occur with both referred and deep somatic pain (Jacox, 1977).

Deep Somatic Pain (related to the wall of the body cavity; parietal). This source of pain includes bone, nerve, muscle, tendon, ligaments, periosteum, cancellous (spongy) bone, arteries, and joints. Whereas the visceral pleura is insensitive to pain, the parietal pleura is well supplied with pain nerve endings. Deep somatic pain is poorly localized and may be referred to the body surface (cutaneous).

Deep somatic pain can be associated with an autonomic phenomenon, such as sweating, pallor, or reduced blood pressure, and is commonly accompanied by a subjective feeling of nausea and faintness. Pain associated with deep somatic lesions follows patterns that relate to the embryologic development of the musculoskeletal system (Hertling and Kessler, 1990).

Visceral Pain (related to internal organs). This source of pain includes all body organs located in the trunk or abdomen, such as the organs of the respiratory, digestive, urogenital, and endocrine systems, as well as the spleen, the heart, and the great vessels. The site of pain corresponds to dermatomes from which the diseased organ receives its innervation (see Fig. 6–3).

Pain is not well localized because innervation of the viscera is multisegmental with few nerve endings. Additionally, although the viscera experience pain, the visceral pleura (the membrane enveloping the organs) is insensitive to pain. It is possible for a client to have extensive disease without pain until the disease progresses enough to involve the parietal pleura (Bauwens and Paine, 1983; Ridge and Way, 1993; Travell and Simons, 1983).

Visceral disease of the abdomen and

pelvis is more likely to refer pain to the back, whereas intrathoracic disease refers pain to the shoulder(s). Visceral pain rarely occurs without associated signs and symptoms, although the client may not recognize the correlation. Careful questioning will usually elicit a systemic pattern of symptoms. Back or shoulder range of motion is *usually* full and painless in the presence of visceral pain.

Referred Pain (related to a remote origin). This source of pain includes all cutaneous, deep somatic, and visceral structures. It may occur in addition to or in the absence of deep somatic and true visceral pain. Referred pain is well localized (i.e., the client can point directly to the area that hurts), but it occurs in remote areas supplied by the same neurosegment that supplies the diseased organ by way of shared central pathways for afferent neurons. Referred pain occurs usually when the painful stimulus is sufficiently intense or when the pain threshold of an organ has been lowered by disease (Blacklow, 1983). Referred pain can occur alone without accompanying visceral pain, but usually visceral pain precedes the development of referred pain when an organ is involved.

TYPES OF PAIN
(Engel, 1983; Kirkaldy-Willis, 1983)

Body activities and physiologic processes serve to modify pain by increasing or decreasing afferent activity. These relationships are helpful in identifying the site and nature (i.e., musculoskeletal or potentially systemic) of the pathologic process responsible for the pain.

Muscular Pain. Muscular pain is intensified by the use of the muscle as well as by mechanical forces, such as pressure or stretch. When pain is due to ischemia, which is characteristic of intermittent claudication, there is a direct relationship between the degree of circulatory insufficiency and muscle work.

The interval between the beginning of muscle contraction and the onset of pain depends on how long it takes for hypoxic products of muscle metabolism to accumulate and exceed the threshold of receptor response. Therefore, pain from an ischemic muscle builds up with the use of the muscle and subsides with rest. The use of movable skeletal parts, including bones, joints, bursae, and tendons, gives rise to pain; resting these parts brings relief.

Heart Pain. Heart pain, a consequence of muscle ischemia, correlates with metabolic demand. With coronary insufficiency (angina pectoris), pain may develop when the work of the heart increases, such as with exertion, cold, or emotion, and subsides with rest and relaxation. Pain from the mediastinum may be influenced by the activity of neighboring moving parts: esophagus (swallowing), musculoskeletal structures (movement), or aorta (increased systolic thrust).

Arterial, Pleural, Tracheal Pain. Pain arising from arteries, as with arteritis (inflammation of an artery), migraine, and vascular headaches, increases with systolic impulse so that any process associated with increased systolic pressure, such as exercise, fever, alcohol consumption, or bending over, may intensify the already throbbing pain. Pain from the pleura, as well as from the trachea, correlates with respiratory movements.

Gastrointestinal, Visceral Pain. Pain arising from the gastrointestinal tract tends to increase with peristaltic activity, particularly if there is any obstruction to forward progress. The pain increases with ingestion and may lessen with fasting or after emptying the involved segment (vomiting or bowel movement). When hollow viscera, such as the liver, kidneys, spleen, and pancreas, are distended, body positions or movements that increase intra-abdominal pressure may intensify the pain, whereas positions that reduce pressure or support the structure may ease the pain.

For example, the client with an acutely

distended gallbladder may slightly flex the trunk. With pain arising from a tense, swollen kidney (or distended renal pelvis), the client flexes the trunk and tilts toward the involved side; with pancreatic pain, the client may sit up and lean forward or lie down with the knees drawn up to the chest.

Pain may occur secondary to the effect of gastric acid on the esophagus, stomach, or duodenum. This pain is relieved by the presence of food or by other neutralizing material in the stomach, and the pain is intensified when the stomach is empty and secreting acid. In these cases, it is important to ask the client about the effect of eating on musculoskeletal pain: whether the pain increases, decreases, or stays the same after eating.

Referred Pain. Referred pain is pain that is experienced at a site other than the actual site that is stimulated, but in tissues supplied by the same or adjacent neural segments. It does not follow normal anatomic pathways and is perceived by the client in an area far removed from the site of the lesion, because the sensory pathways are distorted. The borders of the area of referred pain are not sharply demarcated. There is local tenderness in the tissues of the referred pain area, but there is no objective sensory deficit (Zohn and Mennell, 1988).

There are numerous theories regarding the mechanism by which referred pain develops. However it occurs, it is known that continuous irritation of pain receptor systems in a particular tissue (e.g., posterior joint capsule) creates a state of hyperexcitability in related nerve cells in the dorsal horn of the spinal cord. After this, afferent input from receptors in other segmentally related tissues gives rise to pain in these tissues. Referred pain is often associated with muscle hypertonus over the referred area of pain.

Myofascial Pain. Pain and dysfunction of myofascial tissues is the subject of two extensive volumes to which the reader is referred for more information (Travell and Simons, 1983; Travell and Simons, 1992).

Myofascial pain syndrome is synonymous with *myofascial syndrome* and *myofasciitis.* All terms refer to pain and/or autonomic phenomena referred from active myofascial trigger points with associated dysfunction. A myofascial trigger point is a hyperirritable spot, usually within a taut band of skeletal muscle or in the muscle's fascia. These points are painful on compression and give rise to characteristic referred pain, tenderness, and autonomic phenomena such as sweating, nausea, and vomiting (Travell and Simons, 1983).

The term *posttraumatic hyperirritability syndrome* was introduced to identify a limited number of cases of myofascial pain with marked hyperirritability of the sensory nervous system. This syndrome follows a major trauma, such as an automobile accident, a fall, or a severe blow to the body that is apparently sufficient to injure the sensory modulation mechanisms of the spinal cord or brain stem (Travell and Simons, 1992).

These clients have constant pain, which may be exacerbated by vibration, loud noises, jarring or bumping motions, severe pain (injections), prolonged physical activity, and emotional stress (Travell and Simons, 1992).

Radicular Pain. Radicular (radiating) pain is experienced in the musculoskeletal system in a dermatome, sclerotome, or myotome because of direct irritation or involvement of a spinal nerve. In systemic disease, radiating pain occurs because of dysfunction of the autonomic innervation of the body (see Fig. 6–3).

Radicular pain of the viscera is generally within the segmental innervation of the affected organ. For example, cardiac pain may be described as beginning retrosternally (behind the sternum) and radiating to the left shoulder and down the inner side of the left arm; gallbladder pain may be felt to originate in the right upper abdomen and to radiate to the angle of the scapula. This second type of radicular pain may be characterized by a detectable sensory, motor, or reflex deficit.

Physical disease will localize pain in dermatomal or myotomal patterns, but the client who describes radicular pain that does not match a dermatomal or myotomal pattern (e.g., whole leg pain or whole leg numbness) may be experiencing *inappropriate illness behavior*. Inappropriate illness behavior is recognized clinically as illness behavior out of proportion to the underlying physical disease and is related more to associated psychologic disturbances than to actual physical disease (Waddell et al., 1984).

Diffuse Pain. Diffuse pain that characterizes some diseases of the nervous system and viscera may be difficult to distinguish from the equally diffuse pain so often caused by lesions of the moving parts. Most clients in this category are those with obscure pain in the trunk, especially when the symptoms are felt anteriorly only (Cyriax, 1982). The distinction between visceral pain and pain caused by lesions of the vertebral column may be difficult to make and will require a medical diagnosis.

Pain at Rest. Pain at rest may arise from ischemia of a wide variety of tissue (e.g., vascular disease or tumor growth). The acute onset of severe unilateral extremity involvement accompanied by the "five Ps"—pain, pallor, pulselessness, paresthesia, and paralysis—signifies acute arterial occlusion (peripheral vascular disease [PVD]). Pain in this case is usually described by the client as burning or shooting and may be accompanied by paresthesia. Restless legs are an early manifestation of arterial insufficiency. Pain related to ischemia of the skin and subcutaneous tissues is characterized by the client as burning and boring. All these chronic causes of pain are usually worse at night and are relieved to some degree by dangling the affected leg over the side of the bed and by frequent massaging of the extremity (Zohn and Mennell, 1988).

Although neoplasms are highly vascularized, the host organ's vascular supply and nutrients may be compromised simultaneously, causing ischemia of the local tissue. Pain at rest secondary to neoplasm occurs usually at night. The pain awakens the client from sleep and prevents the person from going back to sleep, despite all efforts to do so. The client may describe pain on weight-bearing or bone pain that may be mild and intermittent in the initial stages, becoming progressively more severe and more constant.

Activity Pain. Activity pain, such as cramping pain from intermittent claudication, may be a symptom of ischemia secondary to peripheral or spinal vascular disease. The client complains that a certain distance walked or a fixed amount of usage of the extremity brings on the pain. Rest promptly relieves the pain. The location of the pain depends on the location of the vascular pathology. Activity pain differs from the pain of spinal stenosis, for example, which may be relieved temporarily by activity (walking) (see Table 12–4).

Joint Pain. Joint pain that awakens the client at night is often due to bone disease or neoplasm. The pain of systemic joint disease is most often deep, aching, and throbbing; it may be reduced by pressure. This type of pain may be constant or occur in waves or spasms, and it may be sharp or dull. On the other hand, the pain of joint dysfunction is invariably sharp; it usually ceases immediately when the stressful action that produces it ceases; it is invariably relieved or is at least greatly improved by rest and is aggravated by activity. The client's answers to questions regarding what aggravates and what improves the pain may be very significant (Mennell, 1964).

When joint dysfunction is the primary cause of joint pain, the clues in the client's history are that the symptom of pain was sudden in onset, occurred after some unguarded joint movement, and was unassociated with marked swelling or warmth. The pain is limited to one joint, is reduced by rest (which is not followed by stiffness), and is aggravated by activity (Mennell, 1964).

Allergic reactions to medication may

manifest as intermittent hydrarthrosis (fluid in a joint), possibly with joint pain. The client with joint pain should be questioned about a history of allergies and recent change in prescription medications.

The development of characteristic features of systemic involvement, such as jaundice in cases of infectious hepatitis, migratory nature of the pain (moves from joint to joint), presence of skin rash, fatigue, weight loss, low-grade fever, muscular weakness, or cyclical, progressive nature of symptoms should help the physical therapist identify joint pain of a systemic nature.

Chronic Pain. Chronic pain is pain that persists past the normal time of healing (Bonica, 1953). This may be less than 1 month or, more often, more than 6 months. The International Association for the Study of Pain has fixed 3 months as the most convenient point of division between acute and chronic pain (Merskey et al., 1991).

In some cases of chronic pain a diagnosis is finally made (e.g., spinal stenosis or thyroiditis) and the treatment is specific, not merely pain management. A constellation of life changes that produce altered behavior in the individual and that persist even after the cause of the pain has been eradicated makes up the chronic pain syndrome (Zohn and Mennell, 1988). In acute pain, the pain is proportional and appropriate to the problem, whereas in the chronic pain syndrome, the pain may be both intractable and inappropriate (i.e., exaggerated) to the existing problem.

Painful symptoms that are out of proportion to the injury or that are not consistent with the objective findings may be a red flag indicating systemic disease. A chronic pain syndrome can be differentiated from a systemic disease in that the syndrome is characterized by multiple complaints, excessive preoccupation with pain, and frequently, excessive drug use. The client may live in a socially narrow world and exhibit altered behavior patterns, such as depression, neurosis, and anxiety. Secondary gain may be a factor in perpetuating the problem. This may be primarily financial, but social and family benefits, such as increased attention, avoidance of sex, and avoidance of unpleasant work situations, may be factors (Zohn and Mennell, 1988).

Psychologic Factors in Pain Assessment (Black and Martin, 1988)

Anxiety. Musculoskeletal complaints such as sore muscles, back pain, or fatigue can result from anxiety-caused tension or heightened sensitivity to pain. Anxiety increases muscle tension, thereby reducing blood flow and oxygen to the tissues, resulting in a build-up of metabolites. This chain of events causes somatic symptoms such as tension headaches, muscular aches, and fatigue. In fact, somatic symptoms are diagnostic for several anxiety disorders, including panic disorder, agoraphobia (fear of open places, especially fear of being alone or of being in public places) and other phobias (irrational fears), obsessive-compulsive disorder (OCD), post-traumatic stress disorder (PTSD), and generalized anxiety disorders.

Anxious persons center attention on pain, noticing it more or interpreting it as more significant than do nonanxious persons. This leads to further complaining about pain and to more disability and pain behavior such as limping, grimacing, or medication-seeking. To complicate matters more, persons with an organic illness sometimes develop anxiety known as *adjustment disorder with anxious mood*. Additionally, the advent of a known organic condition such as a pulmonary embolus or chronic obstructive pulmonary disease (COPD) can cause an agoraphobia-like syndrome in older persons, especially if the client views the condition as unpredictable, variable, and disabling.

According to C. Everett Koop, the former U.S. Surgeon General, 80 to 90 per cent of all people seen in a family practice clinic are suffering from illnesses caused by anxiety and stress. Emotional problems amplify physical symptoms like ulcerative colitis, peptic ulcers, or allergies. Although aller-

Table 1-1
SYMPTOMS OF ANXIETY

Physical	Behavioral	Cognitive	Psychologic
Increased sighing respirations	Hyperalertness	Fear of losing mind	Phobias
Increased blood pressure	Irritability	Fear of losing control	Obsessive-compulsive behavior
Tachycardia	Uncertainty		Post-traumatic stress disorder (PTSD)
Shortness of breath	Apprehension		
Dizziness	Difficulty with memory or concentration		
Lump in throat	Sleep disturbance		
Muscle tension			
Dry mouth			
Diarrhea			
Nausea			
Clammy hands			
Sweating			
Pacing			
Chest pain*			

* Chest pain associated with anxiety accounts for more than half of all emergency department admissions for chest pain. The pain is substernal, a dull ache that does not radiate and is not aggravated by respiratory movements but *is* associated with hyperventilation and claustrophobia.

gies may be inherited, anxiety amplifies or exaggerates the symptoms. Symptoms may present as physical, behavioral, cognitive, or psychologic (Table 1-1).

Panic Disorder. Persons with panic disorder have episodes of sudden, unprovoked, severe anxiety with associated physical symptoms, lasting a few minutes to less than 2 hours. Residual sore muscles are a consistent finding following the panic attack and also occur in persons with social phobias. Panic attacks can be treated with a combination of medication and psychotherapy.

Initial panic attacks may occur when people are under considerable stress, from an overload of work, or from loss of a family member or close friend. The attacks may follow surgery, a serious accident, illness, or childbirth. Excessive consumption of caffeine or use of cocaine, other stimulant drugs, or medicines containing caffeine or stimulants used in treating asthma can also trigger panic attacks (Hendrix, 1993).

Depression. About half of clients with panic disorder will have an episode of clinical depression sometime during their lives. Mild, sporadic depression is a relatively common phenomenon experienced by al-

most everyone at some time, but hospitalized clients are particularly susceptible to feelings of depression and a sense of loss and despair (O'Toole, 1992).

▼ *Clinical Signs and Symptoms of*
Panic Disorder

- Racing or pounding heartbeat
- Chest pains
- Dizziness, lightheadedness, nausea
- Difficulty in breathing
- Bilateral numbness or tingling in nose, cheeks, lips, fingers, toes
- Sweats or chills
- Dreamlike sensations or perceptual distortions
- Sense of terror
- Extreme fear of losing control
- Fear of dying

Adapted from Hendrix, M.L.: Understanding Panic Disorder. Washington, D.C., U.S. Department of Health and Human Services, National Institutes of Health, 1993.

Depression is a normal response to pain and may influence the client's ability to cope with the pain. Whereas anxiety is more apparent in acute pain episodes, depression occurs more often in clients with chronic pain (Sternbach, 1974). When the pain is relieved, the depression usually disappears (Matassarin-Jacobs, 1993). Major depression is marked by persistent sadness or feelings of emptiness, a sense of hopelessness, and other symptoms. Depression can be treated effectively with one of several antidepressant drugs, or, depending on its severity, by cognitive-behavioral therapies (Hendrix, 1993).

Symptom Magnification Syndrome (Matheson, 1991). Symptom magnification syndrome (SMS) is defined as "a self-destructive, socially reinforced *behavioral response* pattern consisting of reports or displays of symptoms that function to control the life of the sufferer" (Matheson, 1986; Matheson, 1987).

▼ *Clinical Symptoms of*

Depression

- Persistent sadness or feelings of emptiness
- Frequent or unexplained crying spells
- A sense of hopelessness
- Feelings of guilt
- Problems in sleeping
- Loss of interest or pleasure in ordinary activities
- Fatigue or decreased energy
- Appetite loss (or overeating)
- Difficulty in concentrating, remembering, and making decisions

Adapted from Hendrix, M.L.: Understanding Panic Disorder. Washington, D.C., U.S. Department of Health and Human Services, National Institutes of Health, January 1993.

The term was first coined by Leonard N. Matheson in 1977 to describe clients whose symptoms have reinforced their behavior; that is, the symptoms have become the predominant force in the client's function, rather than the physiologic phenomenon of the injury's determining the outcome (unless physiologic changes lead to deconditioning). Conscious symptom magnification is referred to as "malingering," whereas unconscious symptom magnification is labeled "illness behavior."

SMS can fall into several categories, and the reader is referred to Matheson's (1991) publication for an in-depth understanding of it. Three signs indicating that a client may be experiencing symptom magnification include

1. The client displays an ineffective strategy for balancing symptoms against activities.
2. The client acts as if the future cannot be controlled because of the presence of symptoms; limitation is blamed on symptoms: "My (back) pain won't let me. . . ."
3. The client may exaggerate limitations beyond those that seem reasonable in relation to the injury; the client applies minimal effort on maximal performance tasks and overreacts to physical loading during objective examination.

It is important for physical therapists to recognize that we often contribute to SMS by focusing on the relief of symptoms, especially pain, as the goal of therapy. Reducing pain is an acceptable goal for some types of clients, but for those who experience pain after their injuries have healed, the focus should be restoration, or at least improvement, of function.

In these situations, instead of asking whether the client's symptoms are "better, the same, or worse," it may be more appropriate to inquire about functional outcomes: e.g., what can the client accomplish at home that she or he was unable to attempt at the beginning of treatment, last week, or even yesterday.

Conversion Symptoms. Whereas SMS is a behavioral, learned, inappropriate *behavior,* conversion is a psychodynamic phenomenon and quite rare in the chronically disabled population. Conversion symptoms are defined as a transformation of an emotion into a physical manifestation. These symptoms may present as hysterical pain, weakness, sensory changes, or paralysis.

No etiology or disease can explain the distribution of such symptoms. Diagnosis and treatment of a conversion syndrome should be left to the management of a highly skilled specialist. However, the physical therapist should be able to recognize potential conversion symptoms in order to make an appropriate referral.

Clinical Signs of Conversion. These five clinical signs of conversion should be considered by the physical therapist during the core interview and objective examination:

Bizarre Gait Pattern. The presenting feature is an unusual limp that cannot be explained by functional anatomy. Family members may be interviewed to assess whether there has been a change in the client's gait and whether this is consistently present under the same aggravating factors. The physical therapist can look for a change in the wear pattern of the client's shoes to decide whether this change in gait has been long-standing.

Muscle Strength. During manual muscle testing, true weakness results in smooth "giving way" of a muscle group; in hysterical weakness, the muscle "breaks" in a series of jerks.

Inconsistency. The extremity(ies) may appear to be flaccid during recumbency, yet the client can walk on heels and toes when standing. A disparity occurs between manual muscle testing and functional performance that cannot be explained.

Movement Patterns. Various movements are performed slowly and extremely laboriously, with facial grimaces. During functional tests, arms wave and the trunk oscillates with apparent tremendous effort.

Sensory Changes. Paresthesia or dysesthesia is a modification in sensation, usually with a sense of numbness or tingling, burning, or crawling. The sensation may be produced by slight pressure of clothes and may be described "as though worms are crawling over me" (Wolf, 1977). The physical therapist should carefully evaluate and document all sensory changes. Conversion symptoms are less likely to follow any dermatomal, myotomal, or sclerotomal patterns.

Systems Review

Whenever a client presents with any sign or symptom characteristic of systemic disease, a screening review of systems should be conducted. Such a review begins after the interview (including past medical history) with questions about general health, the presence of constitutional symptoms, and other questions consistent with the client's presentation. For example, any woman with a past medical history of cancer now presenting with shoulder or back pain should be questioned closely regarding the presence of pulmonary and constitutional symptoms. Any man over 40 years of age with unexplained back pain should be screened for genitourinary involvement (prostate).

Because each organ system presents its own unique set of systemic signs and symptoms, a complete analysis of *systems review* is included in Chapter 12, following the discussion of organ systems.

Signs and Symptoms of Systemic Diseases

The major focus of this text is on the recognition of signs and symptoms either reported by the client subjectively or observed objectively by the physical therapist. *Signs* are observable findings detected by the physical therapist in an objective examination (e.g., unusual skin color, clubbing of the fingers [swelling of the terminal phalanges of the fingers or toes], hematoma [local collection of blood], effusion [fluid]).

Symptoms are reported indications of disease that are perceived by the client but cannot be observed by the naked eye. Pain, discomfort, or other complaints, such as numbness, tingling, or "creeping" sensations, are symptoms that are difficult to quantify but are most often reported as being the chief complaint.

Systemic signs and symptoms that are listed for each condition should serve as a warning to alert the informed physical therapist of the possible need for further questioning and medical referral. Because physical therapists spend a considerable amount of time investigating pain, it is easy to remain focused exclusively on this symptom when clients might otherwise bring to the forefront other important problems. Thus, the physical therapist is encouraged to become accustomed to using the word "symptoms" instead of "pain" when interviewing the client. It is likewise prudent for the physical therapist to refer to symptoms when talking to clients with chronic pain in order to move the focus away from pain.

Nail and Skin Assessment
(Ignatavicius and Bayne, 1993)

Changes in the skin and nail beds indicate systemic involvement and can occur with involvement of a variety of organs. This assessment is an example of signs that should raise a red flag for the therapist. The hands, arms, feet, and legs should be assessed for *skin changes* (texture, color, temperature), vascular changes, clubbing, capillary filling, and edema. Texture changes include shiny, stiff, coarse, dry, or scaly skin. Skin mobility and turgor are affected by the fluid status of the client. Dehydration and aging reduce skin turgor, and edema decreases skin mobility.

Vascular changes of an affected extremity may include paresthesia, muscle fatigue and discomfort, numbness, pain, coolness (poikilothermy), and loss of hair from a reduced blood supply. Clubbing of the fingers and toes results from chronic oxygen deprivation in these tissue beds. Clubbing is characteristic in clients with advanced chronic obstructive pulmonary disease, congenital heart defects, and cor pulmonale. Clubbing can be assessed by the Schamrath method (Fig. 1–1*A*).

Capillary filling of the fingers and toes is an indicator of peripheral circulation. Pressing or blanching the nail bed of a finger or toe produces a whitening effect; when pressure is released, a return of color should occur within 3 seconds. If the capillary refill time exceeds 3 seconds, the lack of circulation may be due to arterial insufficiency from atherosclerosis or spasm.

Edema is an accumulation of fluid in the interstitial spaces. The location of edema helps identify the potential cause. Bilateral edema of the legs may be seen in clients with heart failure or with chronic venous insufficiency. Abdominal and leg edema can be seen in clients with heart disease and cirrhosis of the liver. Edema may also be noted in dependent areas, such as the sacrum, when a person is confined to bed. Localized edema in one extremity may be the result of venous obstruction (thrombosis) or lymphatic blockage of the extremity (lymphedema).

Nail beds (fingers and toes) should be evaluated for color, shape, thickness, texture, and the presence of lesions (Figs. 1–1 and 1–2). Many individual variations in color, texture, and grooming of the nails are influenced by factors unrelated to disease, e.g., occupation, chronic use of nail polish, or exposure to chemical dyes and

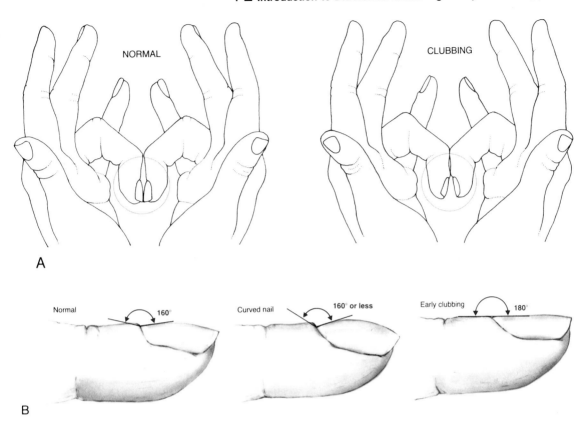

Figure 1-1

A, Assessment of clubbing by the Schamrath method. The client places the fingernails of opposite fingers together and holds them up to a light. If the examiner can see a diamond shape between the nails, there is no clubbing. Clubbing is identified by the absence of the diamond shape. It occurs first in the thumb and index finger. (From Ignatavicius, D.D., and Bayne, M.V. : Assessment of the cardiovascular system. *In* Ignatavicius, D.D., and Bayne, M.V. [eds.]: Medical-Surgical Nursing. Philadelphia, W.B. Saunders, 1993.) *B*, The index finger is viewed at its profile, and the angle of the nail base is noted; it should be about 160 degrees. The nail base is firm to palpation. Curved nails are a variation of normal with a convex profile. They may look like clubbed nails, but the angle between the nail base and the nail is normal, i.e., 160 degrees or less. *Clubbing* of nails occurs with congenital chronic cyanotic heart disease, emphysema, and chronic bronchitis. In early clubbing, the angle straightens out to 180 degrees and the nail base feels spongy to palpation. (From Jarvis, C.: Physical Examination and Health Assessment. Philadelphia, W.B. Saunders, 1992.)

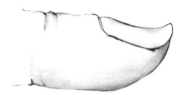

A   Koilonychia (spoon nails)

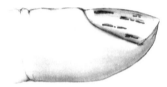

B   Beau's lines

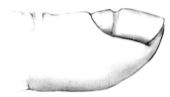

C   Splinter hemorrhages

Figure 1-2

A, Koilonychia (spoon nails). These are thin, depressed nails with lateral edges tilted up, forming a concave profile. They may be congenital or a hereditary trait, occasionally a result of hypochromic anemia, iron deficiency (with or without anemia), poorly controlled diabetes of over 15 years' duration, chemical irritants, local injury, developmental abnormality, or psoriasis. *B*, Beau's lines or grooves. These are transverse furrows or grooves. A depression across the nail extends down to the nail bed. This occurs with any trauma that temporarily impairs nail formation, such as acute illness, prolonged fever, toxic reaction, or local trauma. A dent appears first at the cuticle and moves forward as the nail grows. All nails can be involved. *C*, Splinter hemorrhages. These red-brown streaks, embolic lesions, occur with subacute bacterial endocarditis; also, they may be a nonspecific sign. (From Jarvis, C.: Physical Examination and Health Assessment. Philadelphia, W.B. Saunders, 1992.)

detergents. In assessment of the elderly client, minor variations associated with the aging process may be observed (e.g., gradual thickening of the nail plate, appearance of longitudinal ridges, yellowish-gray discoloration).

Disease Processes

Diseases are presented in this book both by visceral (organ) system involved and by type of specialty. For example, organ systems that are discussed include

▼ *Characteristics of*
Systemic Symptoms

- No known cause or unknown etiology
- Gradual onset with progressive, cyclical course (worse/better/worse)
- Persist beyond expected time for that condition
- Constant
- Intense
- Bilateral symptoms (e.g., edema, nail bed changes, clubbing, numbness/tingling, weakness, skin pigmentation changes, or rash)
- Unrelieved by rest or change in position
- If relieved by rest/positional change, over time even these relieving factors no longer reduce symptoms
- Do not fit the expected mechanical or neuromusculoskeletal pattern; symptoms are out of proportion to the injury
- Symptoms cannot be altered (provoked, reproduced, alleviated, eliminated, aggravated) during examination
- Constitutional symptoms, especially fever and night sweats
- Disproportionate pain relief with aspirin (red flag for bone cancer)
- Night pain
- Pain described as knifelike, boring, deep, colicky, deep aching
- Pattern of pain coming and going like spasms